YOGA TRAINING

A PRACTICAL GUIDE TO MASTER THE ART OF YOGA

NATHAN BELLOW

WHY YOU SHOULD READ THIS BOOK

Yoga is an ancient tradition, one dating back about five thousand years. Learn about the benefits of yoga training and alter the ways in which you live your life. Rev your sex life, lose weight, look to fuel your interior motivation, and finally de-stress yourself in this constantly racing world. Look to the natural benefits of yoga training. Yoga training provides a marriage between the body: your arms, your legs, and your torso, and your interior consciousness. Whereas before you might have thought about these aspects of yourself as different, very separate entities, this book teaches you to join your body with your mind. Meditation allows you to hone your self-exploration; it teaches you to reach for better breathing via your diaphragm. Breathing, as outlined later in this book, fuels you with interior relaxation. It allows you to de-stress throughout your day, even in the hours away from your yoga mat. Yoga postures, brought to you with step-by-step instructions in this book, fuel you with strength and allow you to widen your understanding of your body and its capabilities.

Research-driven information in this book provides you with an outlook on the ways in which yoga affects your interior brain. Boost your gray matter with just an hour of stress-relieving, relaxing, and strengthening yoga every single day. You'll begin to think of your world, your job, and your relationships in a new light. You'll widen your capabilities and maximize your time at work and at home. You can actually build yourself a better brain and teach that brain to maneuver through difficult everyday mechanisms.

Find de-stress techniques that bring interior calm. Learn about weight loss yoga postures that cleanse your colon, regulate your thyroid, and fuel your metabolism. Understand that everyone is wary of yoga failure in the first few weeks, and learn how to fuel yourself forward. Find couple postures in this book that help you and your sexual partner to find greater love and healing in the bedroom. Understand that the world of relaxation and joy can be yours with the utilization of these incredible yoga techniques. When you find yourself standing firm, toned, and revving with extra energy, you'll thank the yoga techniques you've honed. You'll never go back to your previous tense, stressed days. You'll alter your life and your outlook forever.

ABOUT THE AUTHOR

My mission with this is to be able to help inspire and change the world, one reader at a time.

I want to provide the most amazing life tools that anyone can apply into their lives. It doesn't matter whether you have hit rock bottom in your life or your life is amazing and you want to keep taking it to another level.

If you are like me, then you are probably looking to become the best version of yourself. You are likely not to settle for an okay life. You want to live an extraordinary life. Not only to be filled within but also to contribute to society.

Table of Contents

Chapter 1. Yoga: Introduction and Origins

Yoga and its great, classical teachings date back some five thousand years. The ancient need for personal freedom and better self-understanding spawned the marriage of physical and mental exercises. Even the word "Yoga" means: "joining or yoking together;" it therefore merges the strange physical movements of long, awkward arms and legs, torsos, and heads, with the interior workings of the unconscious and conscious mind. It brings you a way to understand your self on both a physical and mental level.

Classical yoga centers on three main body centers: breathing, meditation, and exercise. Yoga considers the body to be the essential instrument in order to operate in the greater world. Therefore, yoga exercises emphasize pressure on the body's glandular systems in order to boost overall interior health. Further breathing techniques bring the idea that breath is the essential source of life that churns the main instrument, or the body forward. Therefore, yoga students garner greater breathing control to increase their body and mind functionality. As breath control and body control come together, the yoga student is able to yield a better mind for meditation. Meditation is essential to yield a silent, healed mind: a mind free from everyday stress.

Ultimate Goal of Yoga Practices

The long history of yoga proclaims that its ultimate goals remain in the following principal meanings:

1. Yoga is a disciplined method that allows you to achieve your greater life goals.
2. Yoga is a technique that allows you to control the body and the mind.
3. Yoga yields a particular school of philosophy.
4. Yoga connects to words like mantra, hatha, and laya. These are related to old traditions that specialize in specific yoga utilizations.

Over time, these meanings have elevated to include analysis of cognition and perception as a path toward omniscience and a way to attain "enlightenment."

DIFFERENT TYPES OF YOGA

Yoga delivers over a hundred different schools of thought.

BUDDHISM:

Buddhism's meditation and yogic principles involve many meditation techniques that work toward concentration and mindfulness. The core teachings align in ancient Buddhist texts and are classically taught via teacher-student traditions.

HINDUISM:

Hinduism's Raja Yoga is defined as the halt of the "perturbations" of the greater mind. The mind is meant to reach toward isolation, or complete motionless. When you are taught to "release all thoughts of your senses," you are practicing a form of Raja Yoga.

TANTRA YOGA:

Tantra yoga is a style or ritual of meditation that rose later in the history of yoga, around the fifth century of the Common Era.

HATHA YOGA:

Hatha yoga is a sort of yoga that focuses on mental and physical strength. It builds postures and exercises that fuels abdomen, arm, and leg strength. Hatha yoga is what most people associate with the term "yoga." It involves physical postures, movements, and breathing techniques.

KASHMIRE SHAIVISM:

According to this yoga study, everything in the world holds both female and male aspects. This marriage yields an equal partnership that cannot be stripped apart. This studies the ideal union of opposites and studies the incredible complexity of the greater world. This Kashmir Shaivism is centered on the emotional aspects of the union rather than the intellectual ideas of the union. Shaivism states that intellectualism is not enough for true understanding of the greater world.

HISTORY OF YOGA

The history of yoga begins prior to written history. The stone carvings that yield prehistoric figures in various yoga positions have been found to date back over five thousand years. This finding immediately disassociates the idea that Hinduism invented yoga; instead, Hinduism evolved much later and brought yoga practices into its religious doctrine.

Over the past several thousand years, yoga has been passed down from teacher to student, through both demonstration and oral instruction. Therefore, the current idea of "yoga" is based on many, many years of different learning and teaching, different teacher-student relationships. Think about how differently math might be taught if it had simply been orally taught to you, and you had to orally teach it to someone else. Remember how different a rumor is after it gets to you after it's been through several other people and their perceptions of reality. Yoga has clearly arrived at its current state far more organically than most teachings, and this is necessary for the subject of yoga. It is an organic, body-centered mechanism, and it must evolve with the people—unlike mathematics.

In order to discuss the history of yoga, it's best to break the yogic periods into four central themes: the Vedic Period, Pre-Classical Period, Classical Period, and the Post-Classical Period.

THE VEDIC YOGA PERIOD

The Vedic Period marks the existence of the Vedas. This is the Brahmanisms's sacred scripture, the basis of today's Hinduism. The collection of its hymns praise a central, divine power. The rituals involved in the text seem to reach past the known boundaries of the mind.

During the Vedic period, people looked toward rishis or

specific yogis in order to learn how to live in harmony. Rishis had the ability to see "ultimate reality" through spiritual practices, and they lived in seclusion in order to continue their intense reach toward the unknown consciousness.

THE PRE-CLASSICAL YOGA PERIOD

The Upanishad creation marks the start of the Pre-Classical Yoga. The Upanishads contains over 200 scriptures, each describing the vision of reality. The scriptures explain three ideas: the ultimate reality, the transcendental self, and the link between these two ideas.

During this time, meditation became a central part of yoga. The Bhagavad-Gita was sung often in order to reach a sort of "other" consciousness. The central idea of this scripture was to move throughout life via benign actions that exceed internal egos.

THE CLASSICAL YOGA PERIOD

The classical period marks the Yoga Sutra, which was written by Patanjali in the second century. It defines classical yoga via 195 sutras. He assigned the eight "limbs" of Yoga, or the eight steps of today's Classical Yoga.

EIGHT STEPS OF CLASSICAL YOGA, AS ASSIGNED BY PATANJALI

1. Yama.

Yama means restraint. Therefore, if one practices yoga, one

must refrain from lying, stealing, hoarding, violence, and casual sexual encounters.

2. Niyama.

Niyama means that one must observe contentment; one must study, remember, and remain pure.

3. Asana.

Asana means that one must continually practice physical exercises.

4. Pranayama.

Pranayama is the essential elements of breathing techniques, outlined later in this book.

5. Pratyahara.

The pratyahara limb means one must prepare for meditation and withdraw the mind from the various sensors of the body: sight, smell, hearing, etc.

6. Dharana.

Dharana means that one must have the ability to hold onto a single thought, a single mantra in the mind for a long period of time.

7. Dhyana.

Dhynana means that one must have the ability to center

one's attention on absolutely nothing.

8. Samadhi.

Samadhi means that one must have a realization of the very center of one's self. One has self-assurance and understanding of one's self.

It's important to remember that modern western culture focuses their yoga-attention toward steps three, four, and five. Therefore, they focus on physical exercises, breathing techniques, and the withdrawal of the mind from the senses in the body.

POST-CLASSICAL YOGA PERIOD

Post-classical yoga verges on the present days. It doesn't work to liberate one from reality; rather, it attempts to teach one to accept the present moment.

Yoga escalated in the United States in the late part of the 19th century. However, it was not well-known or oft-practiced until the 1960s, when the young-oriented hippie culture looked to the East for guidance. The benefits of yoga became understood, and the practice churned in the society, creating greater health and well-being. Even modern-day physicians recommend the utilization of yoga to improve arthritis, depression, heart disease, and several other chronic, stress-related conditions.

CHAPTER 2. THE YOGA BEGINNER: TIPS TO AVOID FAILURE

Yoga can be daunting, especially for beginners looking to maximize their lives with the ancient yogi techniques. Prior to beginning the essential yoga techniques to build weight loss, eliminate stress, and work to better your lifetime happiness, look to the following oft-made mistakes in order to rev forward to your new life of yoga and relaxation.

1. DON'T COMPARE YOURSELF TO OTHER YOGIS.

Your first days of your yoga class—or your days in front of the television instructor—might make you feel a little dejected. Never fear. You're only a beginner once, and you should enjoy these initial days of confusion. Don't allow yourself to compare your body or your movements to your peers. Apply yourself and continue to practice in order to achieve your full potential. Your body will elongate and strengthen with practice.

2. BREATHE SLOWLY AND AVOID ATTENTION.

This is important if you're taking a yoga class. An essential part of yoga is focusing on your breath and connecting to the present moment. However, when you're around people, it's easy to fall into the "dramatic" yogi role. Don't breathe too loudly or portray yourself as "in the moment" just for show. Breathing should be only loud enough for you to hear. Don't allow other people to become distracted by your breathing.

Yoga is very personal. Don't bring other people into your moment; you don't want to be in theirs, either.

3. LEARN TO EAT WELL.

Learn to eat well in order to maximize what you're learning on the yoga mat. As you'll understand later in this book, yoga can rev your metabolism and decrease your stress levels; however, you can help it out by eating a balanced diet full of fresh fruits, vegetables, healthy grains, and proteins. After a tired yoga workout, don't reach first toward a candy bar or a preservative-rich "healthy box meal." Try to live "well" and naturally in all aspects of your life.

4. KEEP A YOGA JOURNAL.

When you begin yoga, you should write down all the "ah-ha" moments you experience throughout your journey. Oftentimes, you'll experience little thoughts, little inspirational feelings when you're deep in your centered, meditational zone. In order to maintain those feelings, you need to write them down and peruse them later. Also, you can plan your next workouts via this journal. If you find that you've been particularly stressed at work, write down the various yogi poses you want to focus on later in order to wind down. This way, you can keep track of what works for you.

5. DRAW THE POSES.

It's difficult to remember all the various poses you have to do either during class or on your own. In order to remember them a bit better and refine them in the future, try drawing them out—even in small stick figures. You can make a short hand for yourself to practice the routines later at home.

6. ALWAYS EQUATE POSES WITH RELAXATION AND MEDITATION.

Modern-day yoga classes tend to emphasize asana, or poses, rather than meditation and relaxation. However, relaxation and meditation are essential in order to maximize your yoga practices. Therefore, after you practice your poses at class, you should try to meditate while walking home, watching your thoughts go by. If possible, you could sit in a park and close your eyes, resting comfortably. Try to take some space for yourself after you've exercised your body in such complex ways. This will allow you to wind down.

7. ALWAYS BREATHE.

Breathing is an essential part of yoga, and it can be very powerful when you attempt to manage your stressors. Breath awareness can immediately eliminate a moment of anxiety. Therefore, you should utilize "breathing time" on a regular basis in order to refresh yourself.

Begin by closing your eyes. Count your breaths as you inhale and exhale. Feel the air in your lower lungs. Begin to feel the tension falling away from your neck and your shoulders. Remind yourself to take short "breathing" breaks by writing small notes to yourself at your desk at work or in the kitchen at home. Just breathing can yield such assistance in the stressors of your day, and you don't need a yoga mat to orchestrate the exercise.

8. WASH AWAY YOUR INNER DIALOGUE.

The voice in your head that tells you that you aren't good enough—yeah, that one. You have to eliminate it in order to accomplish yoga. Everyone has countless doubts about him or herself. Trust that your interest in yoga will override any lack of technical skill you currently have, and remind yourself that your strength will bloom throughout your practices and studies. Remember the scripture from the Bhagavad Gita: "Those who come for shelter, no matter how humble they may be, reach the Path supreme." This means you'll ultimately find what you're looking for, as long as you keep looking.

Chapter 3. Yoga for Weight Loss

Losing weight is a complex battle, one that never seems to end. After constantly keeping track of how many calories you eat versus how many calories you expend, you never seem to lose as much weight as you set out to. This is because most weight gain is a result of interior, serious causes that have nothing to do with "calories in, calories out." These causes can be dealt with utilizing yoga techniques.

Yoga builds the body and the mind with its marriage of breathing, physical, and meditative techniques. When you combine these meditative practices with a healthy diet, you can maximize your weight loss developments and yield a slim, healthful you.

Begin by following these specific techniques:

1. Activate your thyroid gland.

Your thyroid is one of your powerhouses that regulate your weight and your metabolism via its creation of hormones. If your thyroid is active, you have a high metabolism, one that can readily work through the foods you eat and allow you to stay at a proper weight. When you suffer from rapid weight gain, you might have hypothyroidism, or "low" thyroid metabolism. When you work through the following postures, you can begin to correct this issue.

A. Matsyasana, or the fish pose.

When you do the fish pose, you open up the abdomen, the chest, and the throat. This counters the following position— the shoulderstand—because it neutralizes the pressure you've created on the spine and the neck. It further revs the thyroid gland.

Follow the following instructions to orchestrate fish pose:

1. Lie down on your back and extend both of your legs. Splay your arms alongside your body with your palms down to the ground.
2. Next, press both of your forearms and elbows into the ground and lift up your chest. Create a small arch in your back and lift up your shoulder blades. Draw your head back toward the ground until your crown is on the floor.
3. Continue to press your forearms and your palms on the ground. Don't administer too much pressure to the crown of your head.
4. Press down with your heels to keep your legs working on the pose.
5. Hold this position for five full breaths. Release the position and exhale slowly, lowering both your head and the torso to the ground. Bring your knees to your chest and breath deeply.

B. SARVANGASANA, OR THE SHOULDER STAND.

The shoulder stand is very accessible. It stimulates the thyroid and relieves both stress and depression.

1. Begin by lying flat on your back with your arms directly beside your body. Place a few towels beneath your

shoulders, just in case.

2. Next, administer pressure into your upper arms and your shoulders. Begin to draw your legs up into the air. Place your hands at the very base of your back torso, right by your hips, to support yourself.

3. Continue to breathe deeply as your raise your legs straight into the air.

4. Hold the position, with the strength in your upper arms and your shoulders, for five full breaths. Feel the strength in your torso. Remove the stress from your shoulders slowly, moving your legs down straight to work out your abs. Continue to breath all the time.

2. ACTIVATE YOUR LIVER'S VITALITY.

The liver detoxes the elements of your body and works as a cleanser. It processes both your good and bad bodily fats, and it purifies the blood. When you have a healthy liver, you can excel with good fats and repel all bad fats from your body. Utilizing the following techniques, you can maximize your liver's functionality in order to lose weight.

A. DHANURASANA, OR BOW POSE.

The bow pose activates the liver and beats back against both stress and fatigue. Furthermore, it relieves both constipation and feminine menstrual cycle pain.

1. Begin by lying on your stomach with your feet about a foot apart. Your arms should be on the side of your body.

2. Next, fold your knees and grab your ankles with your hands. Bring your head up high and smile to curve your

cheeks and mouth.

3. Keep this pose while breathing for about twenty seconds with big inhales and big exhales. Next, release your ankles slowly and lie back down on the ground.

B. DHUJANGASANA, OR COBRA POSE.

The cobra pose stretches your back muscles and strengthens your shoulders. Furthermore, it warms the inside of your body and activates your liver in order to bring oxidation to the rest of your body.

1. Begin by lying on the floor on your stomach. Your palms should be flat, and the tops of your feet should be splayed out on the floor.

2. Next, spread out your fingers with your palms on the floor and bring your shoulders back with your elbows in the air.

3. Push up off the floor using your arms. Straighten your elbows and keep your legs and hips on the ground. Bring your head high into the air and yield your chest toward the sky.

4. Hold this pose for five even breaths. Release.

3. CREATE A BALANCE BETWEEN THE PARASYMPATHETIC NERVOUS SYSTEM AND THE SYMPATHETIC NERVOUS SYSTEM.

Your nervous system is under continual pressure, especially if you make poor lifestyle decisions. If you sit at a desk all day and breathe in air conditioning, your system might be rotting. Your body is yearning for the natural world. You must relax your interior mind by balancing these two aspects of your nervous system.

A. VIPARITA KARANI, OR LEGS UP THE WALL POSE.

The "legs up the wall" pose brings sanity in a sea of stressors. It calms your nervous system and brings balance to the parasympathetic nervous system and the sympathetic nervous system. It further helps to restore your healthful breathing.

1. Begin by laying out a long, thick blanket against a wall.
2. Sit on the prepared blanket with your left hip of your body next to the wall. You should have your feet out in front of you on the floor.
3. Shift your weight to the other hip and lower your exterior shoulder to the ground. This way, you can swing your legs up onto the wall. Bring your back onto the floor completely and align your spine. Your shoulders should be resting completely on the ground, allowing your tailbone to dip against the floor.
4. Breathe deeply in this pose. The beauty of this "legs up the wall" pose is that you can hold it for ten minutes, fifteen minutes, or a half hour. You can allow your legs to drain of fluid

B. SAVASANA, OR THE CORPSE POSE.

The corpse pose creates an essential calm and relaxation that is necessary to renew your balance between your parasympathetic and sympathetic nervous systems.

1. Begin by sitting on the floor with your knees bent. Place your feet flat on the floor and lean onto your forearms. Allow your pelvis to skirt a bit off the floor and then return it slowly, with an inhale and an exhale. Next, lie down slowly onto your back.

2. Next, reach out your arms toward the ceiling. Begin to rock your body from side to side to open up your rib cage. Place your arms back on the floor, and continue to breathe deeply. Allow your eyes to sink deep into your head, and turn them into your central part of your body, toward the heart. Allow yourself to rest here in this pose for five minutes. When you exit, roll to the right and continue to breathe. Press your hand to the floor and lift your upper body into the air. Bring your head with you last.

4. BUILD THE PROPER pH BALANCE.

When your body is too acidic, your body begins to protect itself with more stored fat. When your body adds even more visceral fat to itself, or the fat in your blood vessels and organs, your body eventually obstructs proper blood flow. The heart overworks and escalates your risk of heart attack. If you are struggling with your weight, you might have a low pH balance.

A. JANUSHIRASANA, OR HEAD TO KNEE POSE.

The head to knee pose brings the mind utter relief and allows the body to warm and raise its pH levels.

1. Begin by sitting at the edge of a blanket with both legs out before you.

2. Next, align the bottom of your left foot in the inside of your right thigh.

3. Reach out your arms and your torso over your extended leg and pull at the foot. If you cannot reach your foot, hold onto your leg or your ankle. Keep your torso long, and continue to inhale and exhale. Allow yourself to fold deep into yourself. Hold this pose for thirty seconds and work yourself up to two minutes.

B. *Paschimottanasana, or seat forward bend pose.*

The seated forward bend pose brings balance to your pH levels and further decreases your levels of anxiety. It massages the digestive organs, and livens up the nervous system.

1. Begin by sitting with your legs together and out in front of you. Point your feet to the sky.

2. Next, sit with your spine straight and inhale, stretching your arms over your head. Exhale from this position, and bring your upper body forward. Reach for your feet with your hands.

3. Wrap your hands around your toes or simply grab your ankles, if you can't reach. Hold the pose and relax, breathing in and out. When you begin, hold the pose for only thirty seconds and work your way up to five minutes.

5. Warm your interior nervous system.

Ancient yogis didn't have to go to hot yoga. Instead, they practiced their yoga in order to heat their internal nervous systems. They generate this warmth through nerve tension and lengthening their limbs. When you create this heat utilizing the following techniques, you can burn the visceral fat and the subcutaneous fat from your system.

A. Anjaneyasana, or lunge pose.

The lunge pose expands the lungs and the shoulders and brings concentration and awareness to your mind and body. It further warms your interior muscles in order to eat up the fat lingering in your organs and over your muscles.

1. Begin by laying with your belly on the floor and your hands splaying out in front of you. Lift yourself up into downward facing dog, with your back stretched out and your torso up.
2. Next, step the right foot out in front of you, right next to your right foot. Bring your left knee to the floor.
3. When you next inhale, bring your torso up and yield your arms to the sky. Allow your hips to push forward until you feel your left leg stretch. Allow yourself to remain here for thirty or forty seconds, breathing deeply the entire time.

B. Paschimottanasana, or seated forward bend pose.

Find this pose above. As you liven up your internal temperature, you can also adjust your internal pH levels!

6. Cleanse your colon.

After years of eating preservatives and living in our nation's environment, your colon is probably clogged with food matter. Your colon can be bloated and contribute to the look and feel of obesity. This can eventually lead to disease and blood poisoning.

Look to the following techniques in order to cleanse your colon.

A. UTKS'EPA MUDRA, OR THE BELLOW'S POSE.

1. Begin by lying down on your back. Bend the right knee and bring that thigh to your chest. Grasp this leg and allow your left leg to linger in front of you. Hold your breath as you hold onto your right leg for about ten seconds. Next, breathe as you bring the right leg back down. Repeat this mechanism with the other leg. Finish by doing both of the legs together.

B. AGNISARA MUDRA, OR THE FIRE POSE.

The fire pose initiates a clean colon. It further eases your stress levels and brings inner peace.

1. Begin by sitting on the ground with your knees bent and your feet on the floor.
2. Next, shrug up your shoulders to loosen them a bit.
3. Afterwards, place the left foot beneath the right leg, toward the right hip.
4. Bring the right foot toward the left leg, on the outside of the left knee. Sit like this, bringing pressure on the heels in order to spread the toes. Extend your torso and exhale while folding your upper body forward. Try to fold from the groin—not the belly.
5. Continue to inhale and exhale for about a minute. Then,

fold yourself back up and remove your legs from their wrap. Continue to inhale and exhale, and repeat the yoga pose with the left leg over the right leg.

7. Yield greater bodily strength.

All great muscular activity brings weight loss. Muscles are tissues that actually eat fat, and when you build those muscles, you can continue to lose weight, even when you're sitting down. Work through the following arm balancing postures in order to build great basic arm strength, basic stomach strength, and basic leg strength. Yoga utilizes so many of your muscles; you'll be burning fat in no time.

A. Pincha Mayurasana, or the feathered peacock pose.

The feathered peacock pose not only builds interior muscles. It is one of the most beneficial detox poses around.

1. Begin by sitting on your heels with your knees far apart. Bring your hands and your forearms together in front of you.
2. Lean your body forward and place your hands on the floor. Allow your fingers to point toward you. Elbows should be bent while the hands and the elbows should be stuck together.
3. Bring your elbows into your belly, and drop your head toward the floor.
4. Next, elongate both legs out behind you with your toes on the floor. Allow your shoulders to round, and begin to raise your head up. Look forward.
5. Next, shift your weight and allow your feet to come off

the ground. You should be on your hands. Note: this is a complicated pose. If you want to keep your feet on the ground to start, you can build your strength over time. Allow yourself to stay in this position for ten seconds. Remember to continue to breathe all the time.

B. CHATURANGA, OR THE PLANK POSE.

The plank is often executed in gym classes all over the country. It's a great, easily-altered exercise to build leg, abdomen, and arm strength.

1. Begin by lying on your belly with your arms along your body.
2. Bring your torso up and lay your palms on the floor. Allow your shoulders to be right over your wrists with your torso parallel to the ground.
3. Perform this pose for approximately one minute, inhaling and exhaling all the time to administer ultimate strength.

8. REV YOUR HEART RATE.

Remember that getting your heart rate up for very short periods of time is essential in order to help you lose weight. This is contrary to the belief that running long distances will help you lose weight. Follow this yogi technique in order to elevate your heart rate for a very short period of time and therefore expedite your weight loss.

Begin by standing at the very front of your yoga mat. Next, perform two sun salutations. In order to do this, bring your feet about a foot apart. Reach your arms into the sky and bring your palms together. Next, exhale and yield your chest to your thighs through a hip-bend. Place your hands on the floor, and continue to breathe.

Next, inhale and lunge your leg back behind you. Keep one foot by your hands. Fall fluidly into a plank pose, bringing the other foot back by your extended foot. Look at the floor and hold this plank for five breaths.

Next, drop your knees to the floor and allow your hips to fall to your heels. Lower your face to the floor and allow your arms to remain extended before you. Continue to inhale, and then bring yourself up into all fours.

Exhale and bend your elbows. Lower your chest and your chin to the floor and keep your knees, hands, and feet on the mat.

Create the upward facing dog by pushing your head and your ribcage up from the mat. Extend your arms as you push the very top of your feet into the mat. Your hips and thighs should spring up from the mat, as well.

Next, fall into the downward facing dog. Tuck your toes and lift your hips. Bear the weight to the balls of your feet, and create an upside-down V. Allow the weight from your head to stretch out your spine.

Next, step your left foot in front of you to create another lunge. Step your right foot into position by the left foot and bring yourself up into your original standing pose.

Do this step-by-step twice in order to elevate your heart

rate. Do this reasonably quickly in order to create bountiful energy.

Chapter 4. Yoga for Stress Reduction

Yoga is the best mechanism to alleviate stress. Some particular yoga positions are essential to relieve tension and provide better restfulness. Find calming, stress-relieving yoga poses below.

A. Balasana, or the child's pose.

The child's pose brings infinite calm in its restful state. It eases both anxiety and stress while stretching the spine. Furthermore, it revs both the nervous system and the lymphatic system.

1. Begin by sitting on your heels with your back straight.
2. Net, roll your torso from your groin and yield your forehead directly to the ground.
3. Continue to breathe deeply as you lower your chest to the ground. Extend the spine and work through twenty inhales and exhales.

B. Setu Bandha Sarvangasana, or bridge pose.

The bridge pose brings a gentle stretch to the spine and the legs. The posture alleviates both tension and stress and has been shown to decrease backaches, insomnia, and headaches. It is known to be beneficial to reduce high blood pressure.

1. Begin by lying on your back.

2. Next, fold your knees into your body but retain the proper feet distance: about a foot apart. Your feet should be about a foot from your pelvis, as well.

3. Allow your arms to remain directly next to your body with your palms facing down to the floor.

4. Next, inhale and slowly lift your lower back, your middle back, and your upper back. Roll in your shoulders and touch your chest to your chin—not the other way around.

5. Continue to breathe easily. Hold the pose for about two minutes and then gently release the pose with a long exhale.

C. Uttanasana, or standing forward bend pose.

This pose is often utilized as a transition between the various poses; however, it provides many anti-stress components in and of itself. The pose stretches the hips, the thighs, and the hamstrings. As it releases your body's tension, it reduces your fatigue, your stress, and your mild depression.

1. Begin by standing straight up and down with your feet about a foot apart and your hands on your hips. This is referred to as "Mountain Pose."

2. Give a deep exhale as you bend forward. Bend at the hips and lengthen your spine as you move down.

3. Next, bend your elbows. Hold onto each elbow with your other hand, and allow the top of your head to hang low. Allow your energy to pivot at your heels, and make sure you don't lock your knees.

4. If you can, touch your hands to the floor. Allow your palms to be flat on the ground.

5. Begin to alternate your weight and energy from one end of your foot to the other. Lengthen your torso and then bright it back with each inhale and exhale.

6. Hold this pose for approximately one minute and then pull yourself back up very slowly. You can repeat this up to ten times for ultimate stress-relief.

D. GARUDASANA, OR EAGLE POSE.

The eagle pose is powerful and can eliminate stressful feelings by increasing your concentration and achieving interior balance. It allows you to open your shoulders, your hips, and your back.

1. Begin by standing straight up with your feet about a foot apart. This is called the Mountain Pose.

2. Next, bend your knees. Balance your weight on your right foot,a nd bring your left thigh over your right thigh. Bring your gaze directly to a single point in front of you, and hook your left foot behind the other calf. Continue to balance.

2. Next, extend both of your arms in front of you and bring your left arm under your right arm.

3. Bend the elbows and bring your forearms vertical. Wrap both your arms and your hands, and link your palms together. Allow your fingertips to point to the ceiling, and continue to press your shoulder blades together.

4 .Hold this pose for approximately one minute and continue to inhale and exhale slowly. Focus on the point in front of you in order to stay upright. Repeat this pose using the other legs.

E. CORPSE POSE.

You might have read about corpse pose in the above weight loss section. Corpse pose is usually the end of the yoga session and can bring ready calm. The corpse pose allows the body to trigger its "relaxation response," or a state of interior rest that actually lowers your blood pressure and lulls the nervous system.

1. Begin by sitting on the floor with your knees bent. Place your feet flat on the floor and lean onto your forearms. Allow your pelvis to skirt a bit off the floor and then return it slowly, with an inhale and an exhale. Next, lie down slowly onto your back.
2. Next, reach out your arms toward the ceiling. Begin to rock your body from side to side to open up your rib cage. Place your arms back on the floor, and continue to breathe deeply. Allow your eyes to sink deep into your head, and turn them into your central part of your body, toward the heart. Allow yourself to rest here in this pose for five minutes. When you exit, roll to the right and continue to breathe. Press your hand to the floor and lift your upper body into the air. Bring your head with you last.

F. Utthitia Trikonasana, or extended triangle pose.

The triangle pose is found in the foundational postures of yoga. It provides a full-body stretch and is essential to improve your digestion and eliminate signs of anxiety.

1. Begin by standing with your feet far apart. Raise your arms up so that they are parallel to the floor. Allow your shoulder blades to widen, and bring your palms to face down.

2. Next, maneuver your left foot to the right and your right foot to the right so that they're both at 90 degree angles. Turn out your right thigh and allow the right knee cap to align with the ankle below.

3. Exhale deeply and bring your torso out over the right leg. Bend from the hip. Rotate the torso the opposite direction, and allow your left hip to sway forward.

4. Place your hand on your ankle, your shin, or the floor next to your foot. Stay in this pose, breathing slowly, for about a minute prior to coming up slowly. Reverse this posture to the other side, and continue to breathe slowly.

G. UTTANA SHISHOSANA, OR THE PUPPY POSE.

This alternate formation of child's pose brings a heart-opening effect to your body. It can elongate the spine and open up the shoulders. This alleviates your normal tendency to slouch and crouch when you feel stressed.

1. Begin by resting on all fours and allowing your shoulders to be above your wrists with your hips above your knees.

2. Walk both hands forward and begin to curl your toes.

3. Exhale and move your butt back toward your feet. Don't allow your elbows to fall to the floor.

4. Next, drop your face to the floor and allow your neck to release its tension. Press your hands to the floor and continue to stretch as you push your hips further and further back.

5. Continue to breathe through your back and your spine. Hold this pose for about a minute and then push yourself back to all fours. Continue to breathe and operate slowly.

Chapter 5. Yoga and the Brain

Neuroplasticity, or the Brain Re-Written

The study of the brain, or neuroscience, demonstrates that the brain has the eternal ability to rewrite itself, or re-wire itself after different life experiences. All experiences alter the landscape of the brain and create different "grooves." This alteration affects the ways in which one relates to one's body and one's mind. Therefore, if one understands how the brain functions via these alterations, one can enact positive change. One can actively re-wire one's brain with the utilization of yoga.

Yoga taps into this idea. It is scientific, grabbing at the interior capability of the body to transform and recreate itself. It maximizes the potential of the brain and the body working as a greater unit.

Boost Gray Matter

Chantal Willemure and Catherine Bushnell, both of the National Center for Complementary and Alternative Medicine in Bethesda, Maryland, have utilized MRI scans to analyze yogi brains. According to their research, yogis have more gray matter, or brain cells, in specific brain centers. They stated that more hours of yoga per week brought about a very obvious difference in gray matter. Certain portions of the brain were actually larger than others.

WIllemure and Bushnell stated that yogis have greater

brain volume in a specific center of the brain called the comatosensory cortex, which yields the mental map of the body. With a greater mental map, one has a better understanding of one's body. Therefore, one can actively feel if one is too full to eat something; one can feel if one is too tired to do something. One is generally more "in-tune" with one's self, which is important for essential happiness.

The brain further boasts a larger superior parietal cortex, which directs the body's attention span. With better attention span, you can focus yourself toward each of your goals. You can reach your maximum potential.

The hippocampus, the region that transfers short-term memories into long-term memories and that further dampens one's stress, was much larger, as well. This means that one can handle the various stressors in one's life. Furthermore, both the posterior cingulate and the precuneus, areas that bring one a better sense of self, boasted great gray matter realms. According to the study, the yogis dedicated about seventy percent of all of their yoga practice to physical postures, ten percent to their breathing techniques, and bout twenty percent to their meditation work.

Yoga Versus Other Exercise

When you practice yoga, you feel amazing. You lose weight, you gain strength, and your mind feels centered. You find a better sense of self, and you work to rid yourself of various stressors, anxiety, and depression. Research shows, in fact, that there's almost no difference between practicing yoga and participating in cognitive behavior therapy when attempting to rid yourself of anxiety and depression symptoms. But how, exactly, does it work to make you a happier, mentally-strong person?

Exercise and its chemical affects on your brain are general gray areas in the study of the human brain. However, the neurochemistry of yoga yields some essential clues to understand yoga's anti-anxiety effects. Yoga, unlike any other exercise, releases something called GABA in the thalamus of the brain. This "GABA" is a great inhibitor in the brain; it suppresses various neural activities that are also suppressed with you take anti-anxiety medications. Alcohol mimics this activity, as well. Therefore, when you do yoga, you are experiencing that "sense of calm and release" you feel when you take in your adult beverage. Doing just an hour of yoga exhibits this same anti-anxiety feeling—without the calories!

Furthermore, if you practice yoga daily, you can have a consistent "baseline" of GABA in your system at all times. Therefore, you can feel calm and less anxious every day— even before you practice your yoga. Beer's calm falls away from you, but yoga's calm remains and builds on itself. It is essential for greater happiness.

CHAPTER 6. SEX, YOGA, AND FUTURE YOGA SUCCESS

Yoga has long-proclaimed its benefits for mindfulness and for stress reduction. But did you know it could fuel better sex? Because sex is one of the most beneficial, anti-stress tools around, you should begin incorporating the following yogi poses to boost your love life and build greater couple happiness.

Ancient yogi practices proclaim that tantra yoga, a form of yoga that utilizes sexual energy in order to fuel higher conscious states, can deepen your relationship and pleasure.

1. UNDERSTAND EACH OTHER'S CHAKRAS:

The chakra is a powerful energy center located between your eyebrows, at your head's crown, at your throat, at your abdomen, at the base of your spine, at the middle of your chest, and at your perineum. Begin to touch each other's chakras more often in order to fuel comfort and intimacy. Try squeezing, tapping, or stroking.

2. TRY SPOONING.

Yogic tantric tradition illustrates that spooning brings dynamic understanding of each other. This is because your chakras are aligned: the base of the woman's spice is at the man's abdomen, etc. This allows energy to flow evenly through you both. As you lie in this position either before or after sex, you can synchronize your breathing and draw yourselves closer together.

3. BREAST STIMULATION TO INTEGRATE THE CHEST CHAKRA.

When a couple becomes intimate, the man should touch the woman's breasts in order to stimulate the "heart" chakra. Stimulation of the heart chakra allows the woman to experience greater pleasure and internal heat. The woman should touch the man's chest, as well, to designate his heart chakra.

4. TANTRIC SEX'S YAB-YUM POSITION.

During this position, you'll draw your chakras together during intercourse. The man will sit cross-legged, and the woman will sit on his lap with her face toward him. She will bring the soles of her feet together to allow the energy to continue cycling around both of them. They'll draw their arms around each other and rock their bodies together during intercourse. During this position, it's important to continually inhale and exhale.

5. MEDITATE TOGETHER.

Begin by sitting in a comfortable position, either on a yoga mat or on the bed. Face your sexual partner and hold his or her hand. Lower your eyes and breathe deeply. Continue to utilize your diaphragm. After you keep your breath in your body for a full five seconds, begin to exhale. After five minutes of doing this toward each other, without looking, retain eye contact. Allow your gaze to remain for one minute.

A LIFETIME OF CONTINUED YOGA TECHNIQUES

A lifetime of yoga contributes to many long-term benefits, such as:

1. Increased endurance, flexibility, and strength.
2. Sheer mental endurance that can fuel you through various stressors.
3. Refined and sharpened abdomen muscles.
4. Reduced fat deposits in but the interior organs and exterior, subcutaneous fat glands.
5. Better supported spine via stronger lats and back muscles.
6. Lengthened glutes and hamstrings.
7. Higher amounts of GOOD cholesterol, HDL, and lower amounts of bad cholesterol, LDL.
8. Better sleep and decreased levels of insomnia.

Strengthen your body and your mind with the beneficial, age-old yoga techniques. Lose weight, find your center, learn how to breathe, and create a better, stress-free environment.

ABOUT THE AUTHOR

My mission with this is to be able to help inspire and change the world, one reader at a time.

I want to provide the most amazing life tools that anyone can apply into their lives. It doesn't matter whether you have hit rock bottom in your life or your life is amazing and you want to keep taking it to another level.

If you are like me, then you are probably looking to become the best version of yourself. You are likely not to settle for an okay life. You want to live an extraordinary life. Not only to be filled within but also to contribute to society.

OTHER BOOKS BY NATHAN

Positive Psychology: A Practical Guide to Personal
Transformation: Motivational Psychology: Gain Confidence in
Every Area of Your Life (Applied Psychology)

It doesn't matter where you are at in life. You may have an
outstanding life and ready to take it to the next level or you
may have hit rock bottom. Regardless of your situation, this
book will help you.

This book will help you gain a new mindset about life and
will improve your image as well as your perception of your
self-worth. This happens through different aspects and
circumstances in your life as detailed in a chapter-by-chapter
guide that you can read. Later on, you can apply what you
learn and make these life lessons your own. With this book,
there is no other direction but towards your best self. By this
handy personal-development reference, you will be able to
comprehensively assess where you are right now and find
ways to get to where you want to be in life.

Leadership: Inspiring Others The Way The Legends Do

This is for all the leaders out there who are set to make
change. This is also for all those who are leaders in the
making. We are going to change things, starting today.

This book is made for people who want a guide on how to
discover their leadership traits, and it is made for people
who want to discover what it means to become one. It is also
to make readers understand that leadership in itself is a skill
that is made up of many other skills. Luckily, it is something

that can be learned through process, and this book would show you how.

Reading this book would also make you understand why great leaders of history became leaders. It will also show you how leadership in every part of society is actually part of the humanity's need for such people. Here, you can learn how to bring out the leader in you by assessing the situation, just like how all great leaders did.

Here Are Some Of The Things You'll Learn...

Why You Want to Become A Leader

How to Become the Leader that You Want

Making Decisions As a Leader

How To Win Friends

Bringing the Best in Others

Much, much more!

The Power of Affirmations: Improve The Quality of Your Life By Reprogramming Your Subconscious Mind: Affirmations Book for the Subconscious Mind

You're about to discover how to exponentially improve the quality of Your Life by taking control of your inner voice. Find out how your negative Thinking has kept YOU from living the Life that You Deserve. Researchers have concluded that those with a Positive Internal Dialogue have Higher rates of Success.

Here Are Some Of The Things You'll Learn...

What Are Positive Affirmations

How Positive Affirmations can Help Transform Your Life

Positive Affirmations for Confidence, Self-Esteem, Relationships, Career, and much more.

How to Make Affirmations a Habit

All The Techniques to Use For The Affirmations To Work For You

Much, much more!

ONE LAST THING...

If you enjoyed this book or found it useful I'd be very grateful if you'd post a short review on Amazon. Your support really does make a difference and I read all the reviews personally so I can get your feedback and make this book even better.

www.ingramcontent.com/pod-product-compliance
Lightning Source LLC
Chambersburg PA
CBHW071252280526
45788CB00004B/1688